MW01092833

Copyright © 2019 by Calpine Memory Books
All rights reserved. This book or any portion thereof
may not be reproduced or used in any manner whatsoever
without the express written permission of the publisher.

_____

_____

_____

_____

1.

You always...

2.

You are
the first to...

3.

You love...

4.

You help...

5.

You choose...

6.

You challenge...

7.

You don't worry about...

8.

You accept...

9.

You appreciate...

10.

You encourage...

11.

You are an incredible...

12.

You give...

13.

You answer...

14.

You are the least...

15.

You never...

16.

You have a...

17.

You think...

18.

You hate...

19.

You love to...

20.

You aren't afraid to...

21.

You are
an amazing...

22.

You understand...

23.

You remember...

24.

Every day you...

25.

You believe...

26.

You inspire...

27.

You make...

28.

You have a
wonderful...

29.

You celebrate...

30.

You are the most...

31.

You have...

32.

You are...